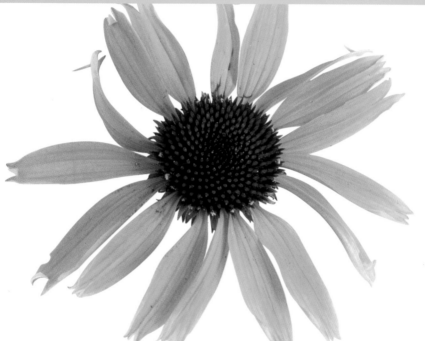

DK *Natural Care*

ECHINACEA

AMAZING IMMUNITY

By STEPHANIE PEDERSEN

DORLING KINDERSLEY PUBLISHING, INC.

www.dk.com

CONTENTS

WHAT IS ECHINACEA?

We're in the midst of an echinacea boom. Walk the aisles of any health store and you can't miss it: Echinacea in capsules, liquid extracts, teas, tinctures and more. Yet echinacea is no medicinal newcomer—the herb boasts a long, distinguished history as an antiseptic and immune-system stimulant. Native Americans used it in mouthwashes, poultices and teas to fight such wide-ranging ills as bleeding gums, blood poisoning, insect bites, respiratory conditions, skin infections, snake bites, toothaches and wounds. Resembling a black-eyed Susan with purple petals, echinacea belongs to the daisy family and is related to calendula, chamomile, feverfew and the common allergen, ragweed.

Although nine species of echinacea grow in the US, *Echinacea angustifolia* and *Echinacea purpurea* are the most potent and the ones most often used commercially. The North American perennial is indigenous to the central plains, Southeast and Southwest, where it grows on road banks, prairies, and fields, and in dry, open woods.

As Europeans settled in these areas, they too sought out the plant, drinking echinacea tea for headaches, indigestion and malaria, and using echinacea poultices for arthritis, hemorrhoids and venereal disease. Indeed, along with its antiallergenic, antiseptic, antimicrobial, antiviral, carminative and lymphatic system stimulant qualities, the herb's antibacterial ability made it an all-around medicinal aid in a time before pharmaceutical antibiotics existed.

Echinacea's most important immune-stimulating components are polysaccharides, such as inulin, that stimulate the body's production of T-cells and increase other natural killer cell activity. Fat-soluble alklamides, betain, caryophylene, echinacoside, glycoside, poly-acetylenes and sesquiterpenes also contribute to the herb's immune-empowering effects. Other constituents are copper, fatty acids, iron, protein, and tannins and vitamins A, C and E. Fresh juice is often extracted from the stems, leaves and flowers, but it is in echinacea's black root that the greatest concentration of these beneficial ingredients resides.

Despite its health-supportive powers, the herb fell out of usage after the 1930s when pharmaceutical antibiotics were introduced. It wasn't until the burgeoning natural health movement in the mid-1970s that echinacea regained favor as a medicinal herb. The rest is herbal history.

IN OTHER WORDS
Like many herbs, echinacea is known by many names. Here are some of them:
- **American Coneflower**
- **Black Sampson**
- **Black-eyed Susan**
- **Comb Flower**
- **Coneflower**
- **Indian Head**
- **Indian Snake Root**
- **Kansas Snakeroot**
- **Narrow-leaved Purple Coneflower**
- **Purple Coneflower**
- **Sampson Root**
- **Scurvy Root**
- **Indian Snake Root**
- **Snake Root**

SAVE THE HERBS

Echinacea is one fashionable herb. So fashionable, in fact, that US sales are estimated at about $80 million annually. Yet this popularity has a downside: Some botanists worry that the current echinacea craze could wipe out some members of the herb's family. Two of the family's nine species–*Echinacea tennesseensis* and *Echinacea laevigata*–are on the endangered species list thanks to collectors who don't distinguish these varieties from the more commonly used *Echinacea angustifolia* and *Echinacea purpurea*. Fortunately, there's no reason to buy echinacea taken from the wild; echinacea that has been cultivated organically is just as potent.

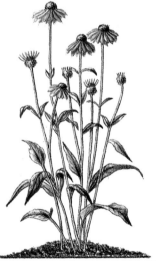

For more information on wild echinacea or other endangered herbs, contact
• **United Plant Savers**
P.O. Box 98
East Barre, VT 05649
802-479-9825
www.plantsavers.org
• **National Center for the Preservation of Medicinal Herbs**
33560 Beech Grove Rd.
Rutland, OH 45775
740-742-4401
www.ncpmh.org

ECHINACEA a perennial growing to 20 in (50cm), with daisylike purple flowers and leaves covered in coarse hair

SPELLBOUND!

Just as echinacea is used to strengthen the immune system, ancient healers burned, carried or scattered echinacea to enhance the power of specific ceremonies. Native Americans not only use echinacea to strengthen their spells, they offer it as a gift to spirits, and wiccans use echinacea to amplify their prayers.

A Native American medicine man performs a healing ritual intended to drive out evil spirits, as depicted by the 19th-century artist George Catlin.

7

SCIENCE TALK

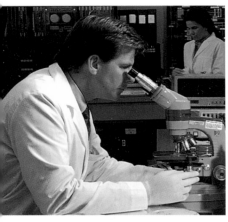

MEDICINE WORLDWIDE
The National Institutes of Health, in Bethesda, MD, estimate that only 10 to 30 percent of the health care worldwide is allopathic, or "Western." The rest of the world's medical care is what Americans would call "alternative," including ayurveda, energy healing, herbalism, homeopathy and traditional Chinese medicine.

CELEBRATING GERMAN KNOW-HOW
Perhaps no other country in the Western world has done more than Germany to further the cause of herbal medicine. What's the country's secret? Commission E, a review board of respected pharmacologists, physicians and scientists. The board was established in 1978, and members spent the first 15 years researching more than 300 age-old herbs for preparations, usages, recommended dosages and side effects. Then, in 1980, the German government upped the medical ante, creating a mandate requiring all new herbal remedies sold in pharmacies to meet the same criteria as over-the-counter drugs. To comply, researchers performed thousands of rigorous clinical trials, resulting in a deep well of knowledge used by doctors open to herbs worldwide.

COMPLEMENTARY HERB
Echinacea works supportively with antibiotics, and both can be used simultaneously. The benefit to this two-prong approach? Echinacea further boosts the body's ability to kill off harmful bacterial infection while diminishing any inflammation an infection may cause.

HOW DOES IT DO THAT?
Wondering exactly how echinacea fights infection? By helping the body to produce the chemical, inteferon. Interferon nudges the immune system into action, stops viruses from reproducing, and inhibits bacteria from producing harmful enzymes.

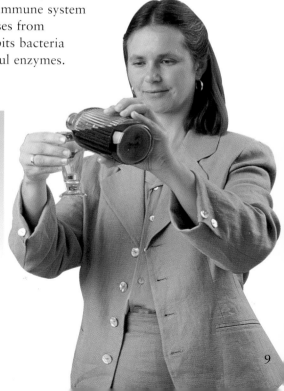

THAT'S A LOT OF PRESCRIPTIONS!
In 1994 German doctors and pharmacists wrote more than 2.5 million prescriptions for echinacea.

9

TREATMENT KNOW-HOW

WHAT TO LOOK FOR

In the market for an echinacea remedy, but you're not sure how to choose one? Here's a hint: The most effective are those containing a high concentration of the herb's active ingredient. Look for echinacea products with 15.0% standardization of echinacasides (echinacea polysaccharides).

ANOTHER TIP

Echinacea root boasts a strong herbal aroma. It also produces a distinctive numbing sensation when held in the mouth for a few minutes. You can test an echinacea product's potency by sniffing and/or putting a bit on the tongue; return any that is odorless or fails to cause numbness.

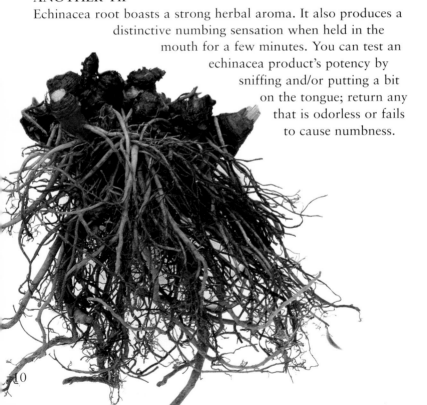

PRECAUTIONS

✖ Do not take echinacea for more than four weeks in a row. While echinacea is an immunity booster when taken for short periods, it has been shown to suppress the immune system when taken over long periods of time.

✖ The doses in this book are aimed at adults. Although echinacea is routinely prescribed in Germany for children's use, we strongly suggest talking to your child's physician before using echinacea externally or internally. If your physician does okay echinacea for your child, we generally recommend halving all suggested doses. Again, please consult your child's physician.

✖ If you are pregnant, suffer from autoimmune conditions, or are taking any type of medication, please consult your physician before using echinacea.

✖ Because echinacea is related to the common allergen, ragweed, individuals with ragweed allergies should exercise caution when using echinacea.

Before taking any herb, ask yourself the following questions:

✔ Have I done any background research on the herb?

✔ What condition am I taking this herb for?

✔ Am I taking other medications or herbs that may affect the herb's functioning?

✔ Do I have any pre existing condition that is contraindicated?

✔ Am I pregnant, trying to conceive or nursing?

✔ Have I spoken to my physician, a naturopathic doctor or an herbalist before taking herb?

✔ Do I know the proper dosages for the herb?

RETHINKING MEDICATION

ANTIBIOTICS: ARE THEY ESSENTIAL?

A recent report published in the *Journal of the American Medical Association* stated that even though antibiotics provide little help for colds, upper respiratory tract infections and bronchitis, doctors still prescribe antibiotics for these conditions. Why? In part, because patients expect their doctors to give them some kind of medication, and many physicians find it easier to oblige than take time out to explain how antibiotics do and don't work. Americans are so enamored of antibiotics that doctors write over 12 million antibiotic prescriptions annually. To learn more about the dangers of antibiotic abuse, contact the Centers For Disease Control and Prevention, 404-332-4555.

PENICILLIN BY THE POUND

Since penicillin's debut in 1941, antibiotic production has shot up from 2 million pounds in 1954 to more than 50 million pounds in 1997. Where is all this medication going? Half of the antibiotics produced annually are prescribed for people; the rest are mixed into livestock feed and used as fertilizers for agricultural crops. The downside to this free-flowing penicillin? New, strong, antibiotic-resistant strains of bacteria.

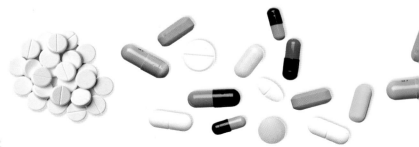

WAIT! BEFORE YOU TAKE THAT PILL . . .
Before asking your doctor for an antibiotic, ask yourself the following questions:

✔ Is my condition caused by bacteria? If not, antibiotics will not work.

✔ Are antibiotics necessary for recovery? If the infection will go away on its own, consider forgoing antibiotics.

✔ Are there alternatives to antibiotics? If herbal or other natural remedies can fight off the infection, consider using one or more of them.

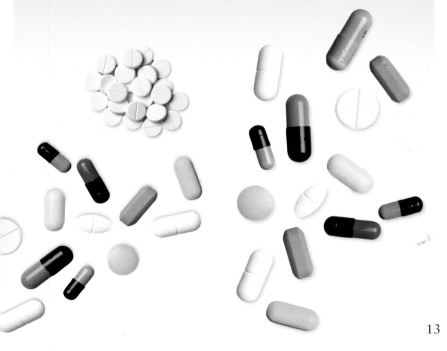

FORMULA GUIDE

Capsules, extracts, teas, tinctures—what do they all mean?
For the uninitiated, we offer this guide to herbal formulas:

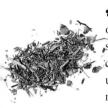

❀ **Capsules.** The medicinal part of the herb is freeze-dried, pulverized and packed into gelatin capsules. Capsules usually contain 200 mg of herb powder; occasionally the dried herb is reinforced with concentrated extracts.

❀ **Herb, Dried.** The flowers, leaves, stems and/or roots of many herbs are often available dried at health food stores and Chinese pharmacies. While these are most commonly made into homemade teas, they can also be used to make decoctions, infused oils, sachets and more.

❀ **Herb, Fresh.** Herbs that are used in both culinary and medicinal ways (such as parsley or dill) are most often found fresh. These can be made into homemade extract, juice, infused oil, tea, and more.

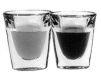

❀ **Juices.** The extracted juice from fresh herbs can be found mixed with commercially prepared fruit or vegetable juices.

❀ **Liquid Extract** (also called Extract). Macerated plant material is percolated in a solvent such as glycerin or water and used undiluted. Generally stronger than a tincture.

✿ **Oil, Essential** (also called Oil). Essential oils are the volatile oily components of herbs. They are found in tiny glands located in the flowers, leaves, roots and/or bark and are mechanically or chemically extracted. Essential oil is used externally.

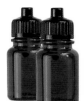

✿ **Oil, Infused.** Made by steeping fresh or dried herbs in an edible oil. After a period of time, the herbs are removed and the oil is used internally or externally. Not as potent as essential oil.

✿ **Ointments.** Dried or fresh herbs are steeped in a base of oils and emulsifiers (such as beeswax, petroleum jelly or soft paraffin wax). After a period of time, the herbs are removed and the ointment packaged. For external use only.

✿ **Syrups.** Syrups are generally a combination of herbal extracts and a sweetener, such as honey or sugar. Generally used for colds, flu and sore throats.

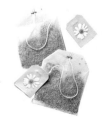

✿ **Teas/Infusions.** The words "tea" and "infusion" are often used interchangeably in herbal medicine. While commercial herbal tea bags are available, herbal tea can also be made with loose dried or fresh herbs.

✿ **Tinctures.** Plant material is soaked in alcohol. The saturated plant material is then pressed. Liquid from this pressing is diluted with water and packaged— usually in small dropper bottles.

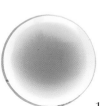

CONDITIONS AND DOSES

ACNE

❐ **Symptoms:** Acne is an inflammatory skin disorder. It occurs when hormones stimulate the overproduction of keratin and sebum, which in turn get caught in the skin's pores, causing blackheads. Often bacteria mixes with the excess keratin and sebum, resulting in infected whiteheads and cyst like pustules. While acne generally affects the face, it also occurs on the neck, chest and back and can be mild to severe.

❐ **How Echinacea Can Help:** Echinacoside, a constituent of the herb, helps eliminate harmful bacteria on the skin, which can mix with keratin and sebum to form whiteheads and pustules. Echinacea's polysaccharides reduce inflamed pustules and promote tissue regeneration. Inulin increases the mobility of infection-fighting white blood cells and stimulates phagocytosis, the process in which white blood cells consume invading bacteria.

❐ **Dosages.** Apply an echinacea poultice or fomentation directly to whiteheads and pustules up to three times a day. During particularly severe breakouts, one can also take a 200-mg capsule of echinacea three times daily before meals; or 1/2 teaspoon of liquid extract or 1 teaspoon of tincture three times daily before meals. As a preventative, fresh echinacea tea or decoction can be used as a toner. Moisten a cotton ball or clean washcloth with tea or decoction, and apply to the face immediately after cleansing.

BOILS

❏ **Symptoms:** Boils generally occur in individuals with weak immune systems. Known medically as furuncles, boils are inflamed, pus-filled nodules that occur when the *staphylococcus aureus* bacteria infects hair follicle. The bacteria then bore into the skin's deeper layers. The result is localized itching, pain and redness. A mild fever and swollen lymph glands may also occur.

❏ **How Echinacea Can Help:** Because boils are contagious, it is important to have a physician lance the boil and remove the infectious pus. The echinacin in echinacea is well-known for its powerful staphylococcus-fighting powers, while echinacoside helps to destroy bacteria and works with caffeic acid ingredients to help stimulate and strengthen the immune system, thus preventing future boils. Echinacea's polysaccharide ingredients reduce inflammation and help damaged tissue repair itself.

❏ **Dosages.** To speed the healing of a lanced boil, apply an echinacea poultice or fomentation to the affected area up to three times daily until it heals. Also, take a 200-mg capsule of echinacea three times daily before meals; or 1/2 teaspoon of liquid extract or 1 teaspoon of tincture three times daily before meals. As a preventative, take 1 or 2 cups of echinacea tea daily.

CONDITIONS AND DOSES

BURNS AND SUNBURNS

❏ **Symptoms:** Mild burns caused by hot appliances, heated surfaces, scalding water or the sun leave the affected area red, inflamed, tender, painful and sometimes blistered.

❏ **How Echinacea Can Help:** The polysaccharides in echinacea help reduce the inflammation and redness of mild burns and promote tissue repair. Caffeic acid ingredients help stimulate the immune system to promote quicker healing.

❏ **Dosages.** Apply an echinacea poultice or fomentation to the affected area up to three times daily until the area heals.

DERMATITIS

❏ **Symptoms:** Dermatitis is a general term to describe any skin condition that produces scaling, flaking, thickening, color changes and/or itching. Such conditions include diaper rash, poison ivy, poison oak, allergic rashes and seborrhea. Dermatitis is also known as eczema.

❏ **How Echinacea Can Help:** The polysaccharides in echinacea help reduce the inflammation and redness of dermatitis and promote tissue repair. Caffeic acid ingredients help stimulate the immune system promoting quicker healing.

❏ **Dosages:** Apply an echinacea poultice or fomentation to the affected area up to three times daily until the area heals. Or gently massage the area up to three times a day with echinacea-infused oil.

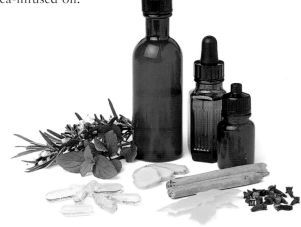

Conditions and Doses

PSORIASIS

❏ **Symptoms:** It is not known what causes psoriasis, a skin condition characterized by noncontagious patches of silvery or red scaly areas that can occur on any part of the body. Psoriasis occurs when cells in the skin's outer layer grow too rapidly. It is characterized by flare-ups and partial remissions.

❏ **How Echinacea Can Help:** The polysaccharides in echinacea help reduce the inflammation and redness associated with psoriasis and promote tissue repair.

❏ **Dosages:** Apply an echinacea poultice or fomentation to the affected area up to three times daily until the rash disappears.

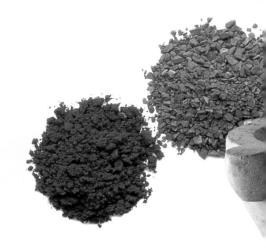

SHINGLES

❐ **Symptoms:** Sometimes called herpes zoster, shingles most often affect individuals with weak immune systems. The illness is characterized by numbness, tingling, burning or extreme sensitivity in the affected area, as well as tiny blisters. Symptoms generally last from seven to fourteen days, but can recur at any time.

❐ **How Echinacea Can Help:** Echinacin and echinacoside have antiviral properties. Caffeic acid ingredients help to stimulate and strengthen the immune system, thus preventing future shingles outbreaks. Echinacea's polysaccharide ingredients reduce inflammation and help damaged tissue repair itself.

❐ **Dosages.** Apply an echinacea poultice or fomentation to the affected area up to three times daily until it heals. Also, take a 200-mg capsule of echinacea three times daily before meals; or 1/2 teaspoon of liquid extract or 1 teaspoon of tincture three times daily before meals.

CONDITIONS AND DOSES

STINGS AND INSECT BITES

❒ **Symptoms:** Redness, inflammation, itching and/or fever at the affected site. In some instances a localized infection may develop.

❒ **How Echinacea Can Help:** The polysaccharides in echinacea help reduce the inflammation and redness associated with insect bites and stings and promote tissue repair. Caffeic acid ingredients help stimulate the immune system promoting quicker healing. In instances where infection has set in, echinacea's inulin increases the mobility of infection-fighting white blood cells and stimulates phagocytosis, the process in which white blood cells consume invading bacteria.

❒ **Dosages.** Apply an echinacea poultice or fomentation to the affected area up to three times daily until the area heals. If an infection has set in, also take a 200-mg capsule of echinacea three times daily before meals; or 1/2 teaspoon of liquid extract or 1 teaspoon of tincture three times daily before meals.

STOP THE STINGERS

Ouch! You've just been stung! Your next move is to remove the offending stinger. For years we've been told to scrape the stinger off the skin with a stiff object, such as a credit card. Yet according to a study published by the British medical journal *Lancet*, if you act instantly, you are better off actually yanking the stinger from your skin rather than wasting precious seconds searching for "a scraper" to do the job. However, if the stinger has been in you a few seconds, go ahead and use your credit card. Hand-plucking it does carry the risk of sending more venom into your bloodstream–and if it's taken you awhile to act you already have enough of the irritant under your skin without adding more.

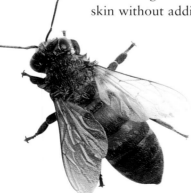

BITES, RASHES AND RELATED SKIN CONDITIONS

CONDITIONS AND DOSES

CANKER SORES

❏ **Symptoms:** It's not known exactly what causes canker sores, or aphtous ulcers, as they're also known—though irritation from dental work, nutritional deficiencies, a poorly functioning immune system and stress have all been implicated. These small, painful ulcers can appear singly or in clusters on the gums, insides of the cheeks, insides of the lips or on the tongue. Each ulcer contains a coagulated mixture of fluid, bacteria and white blood cells.

❏ **How Echinacea Can Help:** Though most canker sores disappear on their own within 7 to 14 days, echinacea can help speed recovery. Echinacoside, a constituent of the herb, is responsible for eliminating the bacteria found in canker sores, while the herb's polysaccharides reduce inflammation and promote tissue regeneration. In individuals prone to recurring canker sores, echinacea can help prevent the frequency and severity of future outbreaks.

❏ **Dosages:** To treat existing canker sores, rinse mouth three times a day with echinacea tea or echinacea decoction. Echinacea can be taken internally to further help healing: one 200-mg capsule three times daily before meals; or 1/2 teaspoon of liquid extract three times daily before meals. (When treating canker sores, liquid extract is preferable to tincture. The high alcohol content of tinctures can aggravate canker sores.) As a preventative, rinse mouth once a day with echinacea tea or echinacea decoction.

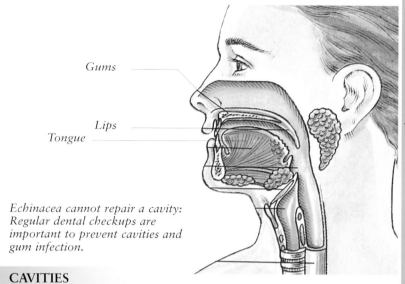

Gums

Lips

Tongue

Echinacea cannot repair a cavity: Regular dental checkups are important to prevent cavities and gum infection.

CAVITIES

❐ **Symptoms:** A cavity is a weakened spot in the tooth's enamel, caused when bacteria interacts with food particles on teeth, creating decay. Cavity signs include a constant dull, pain in the affected tooth and shooting pain in the affected area when eating or drinking something hot or cold.

❐ **How Echinacea Can Help:** Echinacea cannot repair a cavity; a visit to the dentist is needed to remove the decay and fill the affected area. However, the echinacoside in echinacea can help prevent cavities by killing harmful bacteria in the mouth.

❐ **Dosages:** As a preventative, rinse mouth one to three times a day (preferably after meals) with echinacea tea or decoction.

CANKER SORES, GINGIVITIS AND OTHER ORAL ILLS

CONDITIONS AND DOSES

GINGIVITIS

❏ **Symptoms:** Caused by deposits of plaque along the gum line, gingivitis is a painless condition characterized by swollen, soft, red gums that bleed easily during brushing and flossing. If left untreated, gingivitis can worsen into periodontitis and tooth loss.

❏ **How Echinacea Can Help:** Echinacea cannot cure gingivitis—only a professional dental cleaning and regular brushing and flossing can do that. But when used as a companion strategy to professional and home dental care, the polysaccharide components of echinacea can reduce inflammation and help strengthen the gums by promoting new tissue growth.

❏ **Dosages:** After brushing and flossing, rinse mouth with echinacea tea or decoction. Repeat up to three times a day. Or, after brushing and flossing, place 2 or 3 drops of echinacea liquid extract on a soft toothbrush and gently brush into gum line. Repeat up to three times a day.

SENSITIVE GUMS

❑ **Symptoms:** Gums can become temporarily sensitive after aggressive brushing or flossing or after a professional dental cleaning, leaving them tender, red, inflamed and bleeding.

❑ **How Echinacea Can Help:** The polysaccharide components of echinacea help reduce inflammation and strengthen gum tissue. Plus, the herb's alkylamide ingredients create a mild anesthetic effect, slightly deadening any pain. Echinacea can also be used as a preventative before professional dental cleanings.

❑ **Dosages:** Rinse mouth three times a day with echinacea tea or echinacea decoction, until gums return to normal. (If gums are still sensitive after five days, contact your dentist.) To prevent sensitive gums caused by a professional dental cleaning, rinse mouth immediately before appointment with echinacea tea or decoction.

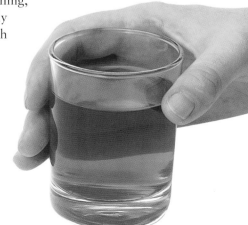

Echinacea gargle

CONDITIONS AND DOSES

ACUTE BRONCHITIS

❒ **Symptoms:** Acute bronchitis is a common illness characterized by inflammation of the bronchi, the breathing tubes that lead to the lungs. Caused by the same virus that causes the common cold, bronchitis is characterized by constriction of the chest, chest pain, coughing (often with yellowish sputum), difficulty breathing, fatigue, fever and sore throat.

❒ **How Echinacea Can Help:** Echinacoside, caffeic acid derivatives and polysaccharides all block viral activity in the body, while another constituent, inulin, strengthens the body's immune functioning. Echinacea's polysaccharides reduce inflammation in the bronchi.

❒ **Dosages:** At the very first sign of illness, immediately take a 200-mg capsule of echinacea three times daily before meals; or 1/2 teaspoon of liquid extract or 1 teaspoon of tincture three times daily before meals. To ease the sore throat that often accompanies acute bronchitis, gargle with echinacea tea or decoction up to three times daily. Continue echinacea therapy until symptoms are gone.

COLD

❏ **Symptoms:** The cold is often called the common cold because it is just that: common. In fact, it is estimated that healthy adults get an average of two colds per year. Most colds are caused by a rhinovirus, although in some instances bacteria can be to blame. Symptoms include cough, nasal congestion, malaise, sneezing, sore throat and watery eyes.

❏ **How Echinacea Can Help:** In Germany, where herbs are prescribed by doctors, echinacea is most commonly given for colds and flu. That is because its components–echinacoside, caffeic acid derivatives and polysaccharides–are especially effective at blocking viral activity in the body. Another constituent, inulin, strengthens the body's immune functioning.

❏ **Dosages:** Echinacea fights the common cold most effectively when taken as a preventative. Upon exposure to infected individuals, immediately take a 200 mg capsule of echinacea three times daily before meals; or 1/2 teaspoon of liquid extract or 1 teaspoon of tincture three times daily before meals. Repeat for up to two weeks.

However, echinacea also helps individuals who have already been infected with a cold. At the very first sign of illness, immediately take a 200 mg capsule of echinacea three times daily before meals; or 1/2 teaspoon of liquid extract or 1 teaspoon of tincture three times daily before meals. To ease the sore throat that often accompanies a cold, gargle with echinacea tea or decoction up to three times daily.

CONDITIONS AND DOSES

INFLUENZA

❏ **Symptoms:** Influenza, or flu, as it is also known, is caused by a virus that is spread between people via infected droplets of air. Symptoms include cough, fatigue, fever and chills, headache, muscular aches and pains, nasal congestion, sore throat and weakness.

❏ **How Echinacea Can Help:** Echinacoside, caffeic acid derivatives and polysaccharides all block viral activity in the body, while another constituent, inulin, strengthens the body's immune functioning. Echinacea's polysaccharides lessen muscle aches by reducing inflammation.

❏ **Dosages:** Echinacea fights influenza most effectively when taken as a preventative. Upon exposure to infected individuals, immediately take a 200-mg capsule of echinacea three times daily before meals; or 1/2 teaspoon of liquid extract or 1 teaspoon of tincture three times daily before meals. Repeat for up to two weeks.

However, echinacea also helps individuals who have already been infected with influenza. At the very first sign of illness, immediately take a 200-mg capsule of echinacea three times daily before meals; or 1/2 teaspoon of liquid extract or 1 teaspoon of tincture three times daily before meals. To ease the sore throat that often accompanies influenza, gargle with echinacea tea up to three times daily. A poultice or fomentation can be laid directly on achy muscles, or 3 teaspoons of liquid extract can be added to warm bathwater, creating an inflammation-reducing muscle soak. Continue therapy until symptoms are gone.

MONONUCLEOSIS

❏ **Symptoms:** Mononucleosis is also called Epstein-Barr virus, after the Epstein-Barr herpes virus that causes the disease. It is transmitted when infectious saliva is spread through sneezing and coughing. Symptoms include abdominal pain, appetite loss, chest pain, coughing, difficulty breathing, fatigue, fever, general weakness, headache, sensitivity to light, sore throat, stiffness and swollen lymph nodes.

❏ **How Echinacea Can Help:** Echinacoside, caffeic acid derivatives and polysaccharides all block viral activity in the body while helping to strengthen the body's immune functioning.

❏ **Dosages:** Take a 200-mg capsule of echinacea three times daily before meals; or 1/2 teaspoon of liquid extract or 1 teaspoon of tincture three times daily before meals. To ease the sore throat that often accompanies mononucleosis, gargle with echinacea tea or decoction up to three times daily.

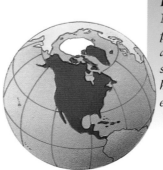

POWER HERB
Nearly 400 studies—performed in the US and Europe—have shown that echinacea has powerful immune-enhancing abilities.

CONDITIONS AND DOSES

Middle ear

Eustachian tube

Outer ear canal

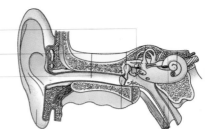

MIDDLE EAR INFECTION

❏ **Symptoms:** A middle ear infection, known medically as otitis media, typically occurs when fluid gathers in the middle ear as a result of a blockage of the eustachian tube (the tube that runs from the middle ear to the throat) or overproduction of fluid in the middle ear. Symptoms include mild to severe earache, feeling of fullness in the ear, fever, chills, nausea, pus seeping from the ear or temporary hearing loss. Middle ear infections occur most commonly in children.

❏ **How Echinacea Can Help:** The ingredients in echinacea work together to increase immune-system functioning, helping the body fight infection. The polysaccharide components of echinacea help reduce inflammation and strengthen infected tissue. In addition, the herb's alkylamide ingredients create a mild anesthetic effect, slightly deadening any pain.

❏ **Dosages:** Before treating children with echinacea, see caution on page 53 and talk to your physician. For adults, put 3 to 5 drops of echinacea extract or tincture into the ear canal up to three times daily to promote healing. Also, take a 200-mg capsule of echinacea three times daily before meals; or 1/2 teaspoon of liquid extract or 1 teaspoon of tincture three times daily before meals.

SINUSITIS

❐ **Symptoms:** The sinuses are cavities in the bone around the nose. Normally, mucus drains through these openings into the nose. When one or more of these sinus cavities become infected by bacteria or

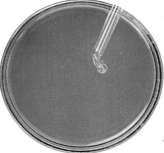

Herbal eardrops can help ease the pain of earache, which is often associated with upper respiratory tract infections.

fungi, however, the tissue swells, blocking mucus flow into the nose. Thus sinusitis is characterized by a feeling of fullness or stuffiness around the nose, pain under the eyes or cheekbones, mild fever and difficulty breathing through the nose.

❐ **How Echinacea Can Help:** The ingredients in echinacea work together to increase immune-system functioning, helping the body fight invading bacterium or fungi. The polysaccharides in echinacea are especially helpful in treating sinusitis. These ingredients reduce inflammation and allow mucus to travel to and through the nose.

❐ **Dosages:** Take a 200-mg capsule of echinacea three times daily before meals; or 1/2 teaspoon of liquid extract or 1 teaspoon of tincture three times daily before meals. A nasal spray can be made by filling a small spray bottle with echinacea tea or decoction and misting the inside of the nostrils three times a day.

CONDITIONS AND DOSES

STREP THROAT

❏ **Symptoms:** Strep throat is caused by the streptococcus bacteria. In addition to a sore throat, symptoms include difficulty swallowing, swollen lymph nodes and sometimes a mild fever.

❏ **How Echinacea Can Help:** In Germany, echinacea is regularly prescribed for strep throat. The herb contains a group of components known as glycosides, which have been shown to be effective against streptococcus bacteria. Another of echinacea's constituents, called inulin, helps send healing white blood cells into the infected tissue.

❏ **Dosages:** Gargle three times a day with echinacea tea or echinacea decoction. Also take a 200-mg capsule three times daily before meals; or 1/2 teaspoon of liquid extract or 1 teaspoon tincture three times daily before meals.

SWIMMER'S EAR

❏ **Symptoms:** Swimmer's ear, or external otitis, is a bacterial or fungal infection of the outer ear canal, often caused by swimming in polluted water. Symptoms include itching of the outer ear canal, pain in the outer ear canal, yellowish and foul-smelling pus draining from the ear, pain in the ear produced by movement of the head, and temporary hearing loss.

❏ **How Echinacea Can Help:** The ingredients in echinacea work together to increase immune-system functioning, helping the body fight invading bacteria or fungi. Specifically, inulin helps send healing white blood cells into the infected area, while echinacea's polysaccharides reduce inflammation and promote tissue regeneration.

❑ **Dosages:** Apply an echinacea poultice or fomentation directly to affected area up to three times a day, or swab the area up to three times a day with echinacea tea or decoction. Also, take a 200 mg capsule of echinacea three times daily before meals; or 1/2 teaspoon of liquid extract or 1 teaspoon of tincture three times daily before meals.

TONSILLITIS

❑ **Symptoms:** Tonsils are lymph nodes located at the back of the mouth. Their primary function is to filter out harmful microorganisms that could infect the body. Occasionally, however, they can become overwhelmed by a bacterial infection. The result is tonsillitis, characterized by difficulty swallowing, sore throat, headache, fever, chills and sore glands of the jaw and throat. Tonsillitis is especially common among children.

❑ **Dosages:** Before treating children with echinacea, see Precautions on page 11 and talk to your physician. For adults, gargle three times a day with echinacea tea or echinacea decoction. Echinacea can be taken internally to further help heal; take one 200-mg capsule three times daily before meals; or 1/2 teaspoon of liquid extract or 1 teaspoon tincture three times daily before meals. Wondering exactly how echinacea fights infection? By helping the body to produce the chemical, interferon. Interferon nudges the immune system into action, stops viruses from reproducing, and inhibits bacteria from producing harmful enzymes.

CONDITIONS AND DOSES

BURSITIS

❏ **Symptoms:** A bursa is a saclike membrane that acts as a cushion between the bone and fibrous tissues of the muscles and tendons. Its job is to facilitate movement by limiting friction. When a bursa becomes inflamed through repeated physical activity, the result is bursitis. Symptoms include pain and swelling in a joint, usually the elbow, hip, knee, shoulder or big toe.

❏ **How Echinacea Can Help:** Although echinacea alone cannot cure bursitis, the herb's anti-inflammatory action makes it a helpful companion to the more traditional mobilization therapy used to treat the condition.

❏ **Dosages:** Apply an echinacea poultice or fomentation to the affected area up to three times daily until the area heals. Or gently massage the area up to three times a day with echinacea-infused oil or echinacea ointment. To further reduce inflammation, take a 200-mg capsule three times daily before meals; or 1/2 teaspoon of liquid extract or 1 teaspoon tincture three times daily before meals. Take until the area feels better, usually two weeks. Discontinue after four weeks.

CARPAL TUNNEL SYNDROME

FEWER SIDE EFFECTS
A German study pitted echinacea against the more commonly used cortisone and prednisone to find out which best alleviated the symptoms of rheumatoid arthritis. The results? Fifteen drops of fresh-pressed *echinacea purpurea* juice three times daily resulted in a 21.8-percent decrease in joint inflammation with no side effects. Cortisone resulted in a 42-percent decrease and prednisone in a 49.2-percent decrease—yet both cortisone and prednisone caused side effects, including adrenal gland atrophy, appetite increase, bone thinning, decrease in pituitary gland function, hypertension, muscle weakness, rounding of facial features (commonly called "moon face"), thinning of the skin, water retention and weight gain.

❒ **Symptoms:** The carpal tunnel is a passageway through the wrist that protects those nerves and tendons that link the arm and hand. When the tissue that constitutes the tunnel becomes inflamed through repetitive motion, carpal tunnel syndrome occurs. The result is numbness or tingling in the hand and fingers and pain in the wrist that may shoot up into the forearm or down into the fingers.

❒ **How Echinacea Can Help:** The first line of carpal tunnel treatment is mobilization therapy, though echinacea's anti-inflammatory action can help reduce swelling so the area can heal.

❒ **Dosages:** Apply an echinacea poultice or fomentation to the affected area up to three times daily until the area heals. Or gently massage the area up to three times a day with echinacea-infused oil or echinacea ointment. To further reduce inflammation, take a 200-mg capsule, three times daily before meals; or 1/2 teaspoon of liquid extract or 1 teaspoon tincture three times daily before meals. Take until the area feels better, usually two weeks.

CONDITIONS AND DOSES

OSTEOARTHRITIS

❏ **Symptoms:** Osteoarthritis, also known simply as arthritis, is one of the most common disorders known to humans, affecting up to 80 percent of all individuals over the age of 60. Caused by simple wear and tear of a joint, arthritis is considered a degenerative disease. Symptoms include mild to moderately severe pain in a joint during or after use, discomfort in a joint during a weather change, swelling in an affected joint and loss of flexibility in the joint.

❏ **How Echinacea Can Help:** While echinacea cannot cure osteo-arthritis, the herb's anti-inflammatory actions can reduce swollen joints, making it an ideal treatment for the condition. The analgesic abilities found in echinacea's alkylamides help lessen pain.

❏ **Dosages:** Apply an echinacea poultice or fomentation to the affected area up to three times daily until the area heals. To further reduce inflammation, take a 200-mg capsule, three times daily before meals; or 1/2 teaspoon of liquid extract or 1 teaspoon tincture, three times daily before meals. Use only as needed. Do not take continually for more than four weeks at a time.

RHEUMATOID ARTHRITIS

❐ **Symptoms:** Rheumatoid arthritis is an autoimmune disease in which the body's immune system attacks itself. Though the ailment is not well understood, it is believed that an unidentified virus stimulates the body to attack its own joints. Symptoms include pain and swelling in the smaller joints of hands and feet, overall aching and/or stiffness after periods of motionlessness, and local fever in affected joints.

❐ **How Echinacea Can Help:** Echinacea's anti-inflammatory action helps reduce swelling in affected joints. Furthermore, one of the herb's components, echnicin, has been shown to regulate immune-system function, which is believed to lessen the body's attacks on itself.

❐ **Dosages:** Apply an echinacea poultice or fomentation to the affected area up to three times daily until the area heals. To further reduce inflammation, take a 200-mg capsule, three times daily before meals; or 1/2 teaspoon of liquid extract or 1 teaspoon tincture, three times daily before meals. Take until the area feels better. Discontinue after four weeks.

CONDITIONS AND DOSES

CYSTITIS

❏ **Symptoms:** Cystitis is an inflammation of the bladder. Commonly called a bladder infection, the condition is most often caused by *Escherichia coli*, a bacterium that lives in the intestines. Symptoms include cloudy urine that may contain blood, frequent urination, lower abdominal pain, an urgent desire to empty the bladder and painful burning during urination.

❏ **How Echinacea Can Help:** Echinacoside, a constituent of the herb, helps eliminate bacteria in the bladder. Echinacea's polysaccharides reduce painful inflammation. Inulin stimulates phagocytosis, the process in which infection-fighting white blood cells consume invading bacteria.

❏ **Dosages:** At the first sign of infection, take a 200-mg capsule of echinacea three times daily before meals; or 1/2 teaspoon of liquid extract or 1 teaspoon of tincture three times daily before meals. Continue until symptoms disappear.

GENITAL HERPES

❒ **Symptoms:** Genital herpes is caused by the herpes simplex virus. Transmitted sexually, the virus causes a burning in the groin area followed by fluid-filled blisters around the rectum and genitals. In women, these blisters may also be found in the vagina and on the cervix. Genital herpes is often accompanied by headache, a mild fever and a watery discharge from the urethra. An outbreak of genital herpes generally lasts from five to 14 days. Once the herpes simplex virus is introduced to the body, outbreaks can recur spontaneously throughout an individual's life.

❒ **How Echinacea Can Help:** If you suspect you have genital herpes, see your physician immediately. Echinacea is a helpful companion treatment for the condition, but it should not replace traditional medicine. The echinacoside, caffeic acid derivatives and polysaccharides found in echinacea block the activity of herpes simplex virus. Inulin increases the mobility of infection-fighting cells to destroy and remove the virus.

❒ **Dosages:** During outbreaks, apply an echinacea poultice or fomentation directly to affected area up to three times a day, or swab the area up to three times a day with echinacea tea or decoction. Also, take a 200-mg capsule of echinacea, three times daily before meals; or 1/2 teaspoon of liquid extract or 1 teaspoon of tincture, three times daily before meals.

CONDITIONS AND DOSES

VAGINITIS

❐ **Symptoms:** Vaginitis, an inflammation of the mucous membranes lining the vagina, can be caused by a bacterial or fungal infection. Signs include localized burning, itching and abnormal vaginal discharge. Individuals who use feminine hygiene products, who are vitamin B-complex deficient, who wear constricting clothing or who are on antibiotic therapy are especially susceptible.

❐ **How Echinacea Can Help:** The ingredients in echinacea work together to increase immune-system functioning, helping the body fight invading organisms. Specifically, inulin helps send healing white blood cells into the infected area, while echinacea's polysaccharides reduce inflammation and promote tissue regeneration.

❐ **Dosages:** Take one 200-mg capsule of echinacea three times daily before meals; or 1/2 teaspoon of liquid extract or 1 teaspoon of tincture three times daily before meals. If desired, douche with cool echinacea tea or decoction once a day.

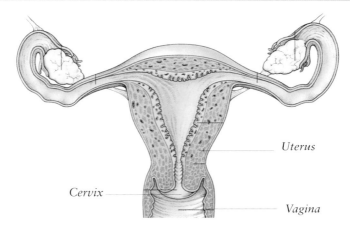

Echinacea is a common treatment for vaginitis. Echinacea boosts the body's ability to kill off harmful bacteria while also diminishing any inflammation caused by the infection.

ANY CONTRAINDICATIONS?

Before taking any herb, ask your physician whether you have any contraindications. This term refers to a symptom or condition that makes a particular treatment inadvisable. When treating most autoimmune-system illnesses (such as lupus and multiple sclerosis), combining the immune-strengthening powers of echinacea with the individual's own autoimmune-system efforts can result in an attack on the host's body, posing an even greater health hazard. Exceptions to the contraindication rule often exist, however, so be sure to check with your physician,

GROW IT YOURSELF

Echinacea may be rooted in the wilderness, but that hasn't stopped it from becoming a popular garden flower. Growing up to five feet tall, the herb displays attractive purple, daisylike blossoms and narrow, tapered foliage. If you'd like to try growing this eye-catching plant yourself, opt for the *Echinacea angustifolia* or *Echinacea purpurea* species. These varieties offer both beauty and a homegrown source of potent herbal medicine.

ECHINACEA ANGUSTIFOLIA

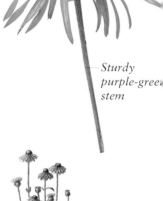

Sturdy purple-green stem

Grows up to five feet

• **Size.** Flowers to two feet tall.

• **Native Habitat.** The limestone hills, plains and mountains of the western United States. Found in a wide band that swings from central Texas through Kansas and Nebraska, as far west as Wyoming, and up into Montana and Saskatchewan.

• **Cultivation.** Well adapted to growing at high elevations, *Echinacea angustifolia* prefers sunny, well-drained, slightly alkaline (pH 6–7) soil. If your garden's soil is low-alkaline, ground limestone can be added. Sow seed during fall or early spring, thinning emerging seedlings to six inches apart. Or sow seed in flats during winter and leave them outside covered with a protective screen. Snow, rain and fluctuating temperatures helps prepare seed for germination—in fact, echinacea requires cold conditioning in order to sprout. In the spring, the flats may be moved into the greenhouse, after which the seeds will finish germinating. Allow the seedlings to develop their second set of leaves before transplanting to the ground. Though the plant will flower during its first year, its root is generally ready to be pulled and harvested during its second autumn.

ECHINACEA PURPUREA

• **Size.** Flowers to four feet tall.

• **Native Habitat.** Although native to the central and eastern United States, *Echinacea purpurea* is extremely rare to nonexistent in the wild.

• **Cultivation.** Easier to grow than *Echinacea angustifolia*, *Echinacea purpurea* is the species best suited to varied growing conditions, including eastern or western United States, coastal or mountain terrain. *Echinacea purpurea* likes full sun, plenty of water and rich, limey soil. Sow seed directly in the garden during early to mid-spring, thinning emerging seedlings to 12 inches apart. Or start seeds in the greenhouse during early spring and transplant seedlings out in the garden during mid-spring. Though the plant will flower during its first year, its root is generally ready to be pulled and harvested during its second autumn.

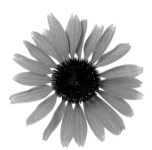

This has less drooping petals than E. angustifolia, *but has similar immune-system properties.*

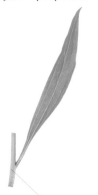

Rough, dark stem and tapered leaf

45

DO-IT-YOURSELF REMEDIES

✿ **Capsule:** Make your own herb supplements by purchasing animal or vegetable gelatin capsules at your local health food store and packing each capsule with 200 mg of dried, powdered echinacea root. **Standard dosage:** 1 capsule three or four times daily.

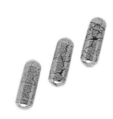

✿ **Decoction:** Because echinacea root is less permeable than the aerial parts of the plant, simmering the root in boiling water helps extract a greater percentage of its medicinal constituents. To make a decoction, place 25 grams of chopped dried root or 75 grams of chopped fresh root in a nonreactive saucepan. Cover with 750 ml of cold water, place a lid on the saucepan, and boil until the liquid reduces to 500 ml—this usually takes from 20 to 40 minutes. Strain the liquid. Use warm or allow to cool. **Standard dosage:** 1 cup three times daily.

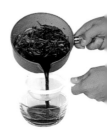

✿ **Drying:** Wash, thoroughly dry and chop fresh echinacea roots into small pieces. Lay the chopped root on trays in a dry, well-ventilated, non-sunny area of your home or place in an extremely low oven, making sure air is continually circulating around the herbs. Or you can use a dehydrator. Drying will take between two and five days. When drying herbs either in a warm room or an oven, the temperature should be kept between 70° and 90°F. Store dried root in a dark, airtight container.

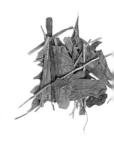

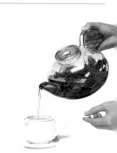

❀ **Fomentation:** Fomentations are essentially gauze or surgical bandaging that is soaked in freshly made herbal tea. The hot cloth is then laid directly on a bite, rash or wound.

❀ **Infused Oil Made With Fresh Leaves:** Infused oils boast the fat-soluble active principles of whatever medicinal plant or herb was used to make them. One way to create echinacea oil is to tightly pack a clean jar to its top with fresh echinacea leaves. Pour almond or olive oil into the jar to cover herbs. Seal the jar tightly, and leave in a warm place for six to seven weeks. Shake it daily. When ready to use, strain the oil and store in a dark, airtight container for up to two years. Can be ingested or used externally.

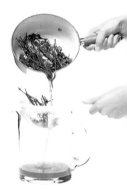

❀ **Infused Oil Made With Fresh or Dried Root:** Because echinacea's root contains the greatest percentage of the plant's medicinal properties, infused oil made with the root is stronger than infused oil made with the leaves. To make, place 200 g of dried echinacea root in a nonreactive saucepan and cover with 500 ml of almond or olive oil. Simmer over very low heat for three hours. Allow mixture to cool. Strain the oil and store it in a dark, airtight container for up to two years. Can be ingested or used externally.

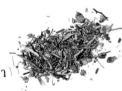

DO-IT-YOURSELF REMEDIES

❀ **Liquid Extract.** Also known as extract. To make echinacea extract, macerate 100 to 200 g of dried echinacea root, or 300 to 500 g of fresh echinacea root. Place the herb in a jar and pour in 335 ml Vodka (37 proof or higher) and 165 ml water. Place the lid on the jar and store in a dark area for four to eight weeks. Shake the mixture daily. When ready, strain the mixture, pressing all remaining liquid from the echinacea root. Place liquid in a nonreactive saucepan and simmer over medium heat for 20 to 40 minutes until the liquid has been reduced by a third. This process burns off the alcohol, leaving the medicinal liquid behind. Allow liquid to cool and decant into several dropper bottles or a clean glass bottle. Standard dose is 5 ml three times daily.

❀ **Ointment:** Also called a salve, herbal ointment is easy to make at home. To create your own echinacea ointment for bites and rashes, mix 1 to 2 parts beeswax or soft paraffin wax, 7 parts cocoa butter, and 3 parts powdered echinacea root in a nonreactive saucepan. Cook the mixture for one to two hours on a low setting. Let cool, package in an airtight container and apply up to three times daily.

❀ **Poultice:** Fresh herbs can be applied directly to bites and rashes when fashioned into a poultice. To make an echinacea poultice, chop fresh or dried root. Boil in a small amount of water for 5 minutes (or use a microwave). Squeeze out any excess liquid from the boiled herb (reserve liquid). Lay the echinacea directly on the skin and cover with a warm moist towel. Leave in place for up to 30 minutes. The reserved liquid can be rewarmed and used to reheat the towel.

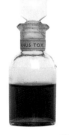

❀ Syrup: Echinacea has a strong taste that may not be palatable to some individuals. Syrup delivers the herb's medicinal benefits in an easy-to-swallow (and throat-soothing) base. To make, mix 7 parts echinacea tea or decoction in a nonreactive saucepan with 10 parts sugar. Cook the mixture over low heat until it has formed a thick, syrupy consistency. For coughs and sore throats, take 1 or 2 tablespoons up to four times daily.

❀ Tea: Also known as an infusion, tea is an easy and common way to ingest an herb. To make echinacea tea, steep 1 teaspoon dried root or 1 tablespoon fresh leaves for five minutes in 1 cup of boiling water. Add fructose, sugar or honey to sweeten. Standard dosage is 1 cup of tea three times daily.

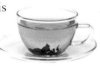

❀ Tinctures: Though not as potent as liquid extracts, tinctures are minimally processed, making them a favorite remedy of many herbalists. To make your own echinacea tincture, place 100 to 200 g of dried echinacea root, or 300 to 500 g of fresh echinacea root, in a large jar and cover with 500 ml vodka (37 proof or higher). Place the lid on the jar and store in a dark area for four to six weeks. Shake the bottle daily. When ready to use, strain the mixture, pressing all remaining liquid from the echinacea root. Decant into several dropper bottles or a clean glass bottle. Will keep for up to two years. Shake before using.

HERB GLOSSARY

After being used for centuries in Africa, Asia and Europe, herbs are finally making their way into American homes. Which is exactly where they belong. Herbs are good medicine. So good that many of our modern drugs are based on herbs' active ingredients. For example, the active component in aspirin is salicin, a biologically active ingredient of white willow bark. Salicin is also found in lesser amounts in birch bark and peppermint.

Herbal remedies come in a variety of forms, including dried and fresh leaves, capsules, liquid extracts, oils, teas, tinctures and more. Doses generally depend on the remedy's form and its potency. Currently there is no US government agency that checks the concentration of an herbal remedy's active

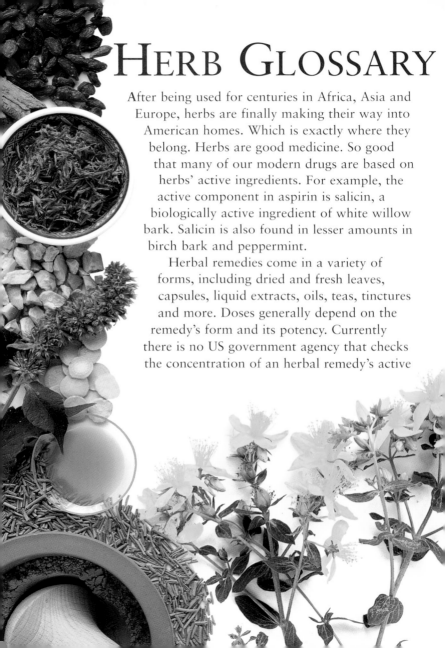

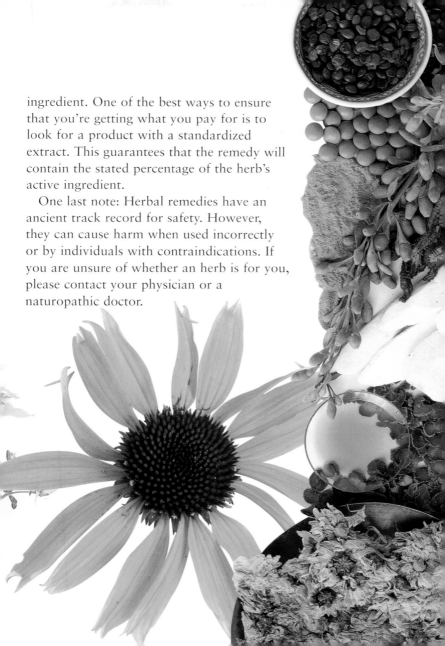

ingredient. One of the best ways to ensure that you're getting what you pay for is to look for a product with a standardized extract. This guarantees that the remedy will contain the stated percentage of the herb's active ingredient.

One last note: Herbal remedies have an ancient track record for safety. However, they can cause harm when used incorrectly or by individuals with contraindications. If you are unsure of whether an herb is for you, please contact your physician or a naturopathic doctor.

ALOE

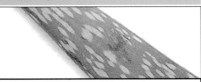

Properties: Analgesic, antibacterial, antifungal, anti-inflammatory, anti-itch, antiseptic, circulatory stimulant, digestive aid, immune-system stimulant, laxative.

Target Ailments: Acne, bruises, burns, constipation, cuts, insect bites, digestive disorders, rashes, ulcers, wounds.

Available Forms: Capsule, fresh leaves, gel, juice, liquid extract.

Possible Side Effects: When taken internally, aloe can cause severe cramping in some individuals.

Precautions: Pregnant women should not ingest aloe; It can stimulate uterine contractions.

CALENDULA

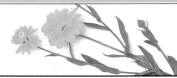

Properties: Antibacterial, anti-inflammatory, antiseptic, antispasmodic, promotes sweating, sedative.

Target Ailments: Burns, cuts, fungal infections, gallbladder conditions, hepatitis, indigestion, irregular menstruation, insect bites, menstrual cramps, mouth sores, skin rashes, ulcers, wounds.

Available Forms: Capsule, dried herb, fresh herb, liquid extract, lotion, oil, ointment, tincture.

Possible Side Effects: None expected.

Precautions: Calendula is related to ragweed. Individuals allergic to ragweed should consult a physician before using calendula.

ASTRAGALUS

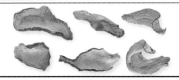

Properties: Antibacterial, anti-inflammatory, antioxidant, antiviral, diuretic, immune-system stimulant.

Target Ailments: Cancer, colds, appetite loss, diarrhea, fatigue, flu, heart conditions, HIV, viral infections.

Available Forms: Capsule, dried herb, fresh herb, liquid extract, tea, tincture.

Possible Side Effects: None expected.

Precautions: Astragalus should be used as a companion therapy to—not a replacement for—traditional cancer and HIV therapies.

CHAMOMILE

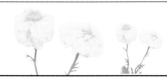

Properties: Antibacterial, anti-inflammatory, antiseptic, antispasmodic, carminative, digestive aid, fever reducer, sedative.

Target Ailments: Gingivitis, hemorrhoids, insomnia, indigestion, intestinal gas, menstrual cramps, nausea, nervousness, stomachaches, sunburns, tension, ulcers, varicose veins.

Available Forms: Capsule, dried herb, fresh herb, liquid extract, lotion, oil, tea, tincture.

Possible Side Effects: None expected.

Precautions: Because chamomile is related to ragweed, individuals with ragweed allergies should consult a physician before using chamomile.

DONG QUAI

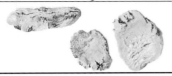

Properties: Antiallergenic, antispasmodic, diuretic, mild laxative, muscle relaxant, vasodilator.
Target Ailments: Abscesses, blurred vision, heart palpitations, irregular menstruation, light-headedness, menstrual pain, pallor, poor circulation.
Available Forms: Capsule, dried herb, liquid extract, tincture.
Possible Side Effects: Can cause photosensitivity in some individuals.
Precautions: Dong quai has abortive abilities; Do not take while pregnant.

FEVERFEW

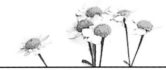

Properties: Anti-inflammatory, fever reducer.
Target Ailments: Arthritis, asthma, dermatitis, menstrual pain, migraines.
Available Forms: Capsule, dried herb, fresh herb, liquid extract, tincture.
Possible Side Effects: Some individuals experience "withdrawal" symptoms after taking feverfew, including fatigue and nervousness.
Precautions: Because it is related to ragweed, individuals with ragweed allergies should consult a physician before using feverfew.

ECHINACEA

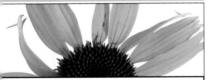

Properties: Antiallergenic, antibacterial, antiseptic, antimicrobial, antiviral, carminative, lymphatic tonic.
Target Ailments: Abscesses, acne, bladder infections, blood poisoning, burns, colds, eczema, food poisoning, flu, insect bites, kidney infections, mononucleosis, respiratory infections, sore throats.
Available Forms: Capsule, dried herb, liquid extract, tea, tincture.
Possible Side Effects: High doses can cause dizziness and nausea.
Precautions: Do not take echinacea for more than four weeks in a row.

GARLIC

Properties: Antibacterial, anticoagulant, antifungal, anti-inflammatory, antiviral, cholesterol reducer, digestive aid, immune-system stimulant, worm-fighting.
Target Ailments: Arteriosclerosis, arthritis, bladder infections, colds, digestive upset, flu, heart conditions, high blood pressure, high blood cholesterol, viral infections.
Available Forms: Capsule, fresh cloves, liquid extract, oil, tincture.
Possible Side Effects: Can cause upset stomach.
Precautions: While garlic is safe taken in culinary doses, individuals on anticoagulant medications should consult their doctors before supplementing their diet with garlic.

GINGER

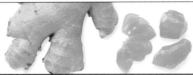

Properties: Antibacterial, anticoagulant, antinausea, antispasmodic, antiviral, carminative, digestive aid, expectorant, immune-system stimulant, muscle relaxant.
Target Ailments: Burns, colds, flu, high blood pressure, high cholesterol, liver conditions, intestinal gas, menstrual cramps, motion sickness, nausea, stomachaches.
Available Forms: Capsule, dried root, tea.
Possible Side Effects: Heartburn.
Precautions: While ginger is safe in culinary doses, individuals who suffer from a blood-clotting disorder or are on anticoagulant medication should consult a physician before supplementing their diet with the herb.

GINSENG

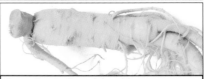

Properties: Antibacterial, antidepressant, immune-system stimulant, stimulant.
Target Ailments: Colds, depression, fatigue, flu, impaired immune system, respiratory conditions, stress.
Available Forms: Capsule, dried root, fresh root, liquid extract, tincture, tea.
Possible Side Effects: Large doses of ginseng can cause breast soreness, headaches or skin rashes in some individuals.
Precautions: Ginseng can aggravate existing heart palpitations or high blood pressure.

GINKGO BILOBA

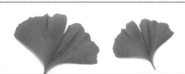

Properties: Antibacterial, anti-inflammatory, antioxidant, circulatory stimulant, vasodilator.
Target Ailments: Clotting disorders, dementia, depression, headaches, hearing loss, Raynaud's syndrome, tinnitus, vascular diseases, vertigo.
Available Forms: Capsule, dry herb, liquid extract, tincture, tea.
Possible Side Effects: Diarrhea, irritability, nausea, restlessness.
Precautions: Do not use ginkgo biloba if you have a blood-clotting disorder like hemophilia or are taking anticoagulant medications.

GOLDENSEAL

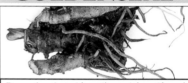

Properties: Antacid, antibacterial, antifungal, anti-inflammatory, antiseptic, astringent, digestive aid, stimulant.
Target Ailments: Canker sores, contact dermatitis, diarrhea, eczema, food poisoning.
Available Forms: Capsule, dry herb, liquid extract, tea, tincture.
Possible Side Effects: In high doses, goldenseal can cause diarrhea and nausea and can irritate the skin, mouth and throat.
Precautions: Because of its high cost, many manufacturers adulterate preparations with less costly herbs, such as barberry, yellow dock or bloodroot, some of which can cause unwanted reactions when taken in high doses.

KAVA

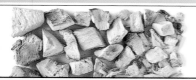

Properties: Antidepressant, antispasmodic, aphrodisiac, diuretic, muscle relaxant, sedative.

Target Ailments: Anxiety, colds, depression, menstrual conditions, muscle cramps, respiratory tract conditions, stress.

Available Forms: Capsule, dried herb, liquid extract, tea, tincture.

Possible Side Effects: Allergic skin reactions, muscle weakness, red eyes, sleepiness.

Precautions: In high doses, kava can impair motor reflexes and cause breathing problems.

MILK THISTLE

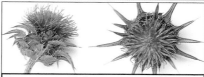

Properties: Anti-inflammatory, antioxidant, digestive aid, immune-system stimulant.

Target Ailments: inflammation of the gallbladder duct, hepatitis, liver conditions, poisoning from ingestion of the death cup mushroom, psoriasis.

Available Forms: Capsule, dried herb, fresh herb, powder, tea, tincture.

Possible Side Effects: Milk thistle can cause mild diarrhea when taken in large doses.

Precautions: If you think you have a liver disorder, seek medical advice before taking this herb.

LAVENDER

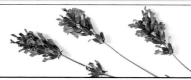

Properties: Antibacterial, antidepressant, antiseptic, antispasmodic, carminative, circulatory stimulant, digestive aid, diuretic, sedative.

Target Ailments: Anxiety, depression, headache, insomnia, intestinal gas, nausea, tension.

Available Forms: Capsule, dried herb, fresh herb, oil, tincture.

Possible Side Effects: Lavender products can cause skin irritation in sensitive individuals.

Precautions: Lavender oil is poisonous when ingested internally.

PARSLEY

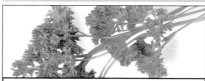

Properties: Antiseptic, antispasmodic, digestive aid, diuretic, laxative, muscle relaxant.

Target Ailments: Colds, congestion, fever, flu, indigestion, irregular menstruation, premenstrual syndrome, stimulating the production of breast milk, stomachaches.

Available Forms: Capsule, dried herb, fresh herb, liquid extract, oil, tea, tincture.

Possible Side Effects: Can cause photosensitivity in some individuals.

Precautions: Parsley should not be ingested in large amounts or used externally during pregnancy; it contains compounds that may stimulate uterine muscles and possibly cause miscarriage.

PEPPERMINT

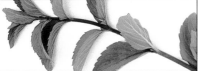

Properties: Antacid, antibacterial, antidepressant, antispasmodic, carminatve, expectorant, muscle relaxant, promotes sweating.
Target Ailments: Anxiety, colds, fever, flu, insomnia, intestinal gas, itching, migraines, morning sickness, motion sickness, nausea.
Available Forms: Capsule, dried herb, fresh herb, lozenge, oil, ointment, tea, tincture.
Possible Side Effects: When applied externally, peppermint products can cause skin reactions in sensitive individuals.
Precautions: If you have a hiatal hernia, talk to your doctor before using peppermint products externally or internally; the oil in the plant can exacerbate symptoms.

SAGE

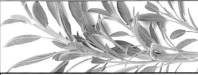

Properties: Antiseptic, anti-inflammatory, antioxidant, antispasmodic, astringent, bile stimulant, carminative, reduces perspiration.
Target Ailments: Excess intestinal gas, insect bites, menopausal night sweats, poor circulation, reduces milk flow at weaning, sore throat, stomachaches, mouth ulcers.
Available Forms: Capsule, dried herb, fresh herb, liquid extract, oil, tincture.
Possible Side Effects: Sage tea may cause inflammation of the lips and/or tongue in some individuals.
Precautions: Do not ingest pure sage oil; it is toxic when taken internally.

ROSEMARY

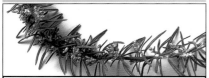

Properties: Antibacterial, antidepressant, anti-inflammatory, antiseptic, carminative, circultory stimulant.
Target Ailments: Bad breath, dandruff, depression, eczema, headaches, indigestion, joint inflammation, mouth and throat infections, muscle pain, psoriasis, rheumatoid arthritis.
Available Forms: Dried herb, fresh herb, ingestible rosemary-flavored oil, oil, ointment, tea, tincture.
Possible Side Effects: Rosemary oil can cause skin inflammation and/or dermatitis.
Precautions: Do not mistake regular rosemary oil for ingestible rosemary-flavored oil.

SAW PALMETTO

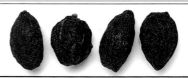

Properties: Antiallergenic, anti-inflammatory, diuretic, immune-boosting.
Target Ailments: Asthma, benign prostatic hyperplasia, bronchitis, colds, cystitis, impotence, male infertility, nasal congestion, sinus conditions, sore throats.
Available Forms: Capsule, dried herb, fresh herb, liquid extract, oil, tea, tincture.
Possible Side Effects: Can cause diarrhea if taken in large doses.
Precautions: Due to its hormonal actions, saw palmetto may interact negatively with prostate medicines or hormonal treatments such as estrogen replacement therapy, possibly canceling out their effectiveness.

ST. JOHN'S WORT

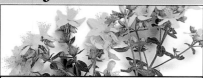

Properties: Analgesic, antibacterial, anti-depressant, anti-inflammatory, antiviral, astringent.

Target Ailments: Attention deficit disorder, anxiety, bacterial infections, burns, carpal tunnel syndrome, depression, HIV, menopause.

Available Forms: Capsule, dried herb, liquid extract, oil, ointment, tea, tincture.

Possible Side Effects: Gastrointestinal upset, headaches, photosensitivity, stiff neck.

Precautions: Avoid foods containing the amino acid tyramine when taking St. John's wort; the interaction of the two can cause an increase in blood pressure. Foods with tyramine include beer, coffee, wine, chocolate and fava beans.

WILD YAM

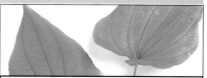

Properties: Analgesic, anti-inflammatory, antispasmodic, expectorant, muscle relaxant, promotes sweating.

Target Ailments: Menopause, menstrual cramps, morning sickness, nausea, rheumatoid arthritis, urinary tract infections.

Available Forms: Capsule, cream, dried root, liquid extract, oil, powder, tincture.

Possible Side Effects: Can cause vomiting in large doses.

Precautions: Individuals who are suffering from a hormone-sensitive cancer, such as breast or uterine cancer, should avoid wild yam. Some experts believe that the herb can encourage the growth of cancer cells.

VALERIAN

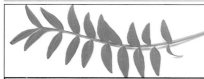

Properties: Analgesic, antibacterial, antispasmodic, carminative, reduces blood pressure, sedative, tranquilizer.

Target Ailments: Brachial spasm, high blood pressure, insomnia, palpitations, menstrual pain, migraines, muscle cramps, nervousness, tension headaches, wounds.

Available Forms: Capsules, dried herb, liquid extract, oil, teas, tincture.

Possible Side Effects: Headaches with prolonged use.

Precautions: Do not take with other sedatives, including alcohol. Do not drive or operate machinery after taking valerian.

YARROW

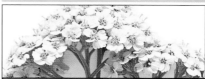

Properties: Antibacterial, anti-inflammatory, antispasmodic, blood coagulator, bile stimulating, immune-system stimulant, promotes sweating, sedative.

Target Ailments: Anxiety, colds and flu, cystitis, digestive disorders, menstrual cramps, minor wounds, nosebleeds, poor circulation, skin rashes.

Available Forms: Dried herb, capsule, liquid extract, oil, tea, tincture.

Possible Side Effects: Diarrhea, skin rash.

Precautions: Yarrow is related to ragweed and can cause an allergic reaction in individuals with ragweed allergies. Do not take if pregnant; it can induce miscarriage.

HERBAL TERMS

You're thumbing through the latest herbal therapy book when you run smack into the word "emmenagogue." Or perhaps you get tangled on "oxytocic." For anyone who's ever been stopped by an unfamiliar alternative medical term, we offer the following list:

Adaptogenic: Increases resistance and resilience to stress. Supports adrenal gland functioning.
Alterative: Blood purifier that improves the condition of the blood, improves digestion, and increases the appetite. Used to treat conditions arising from or causing toxicity.
Analgesic: Herb that relieves pain either by relaxing muscles or reducing pain signals to the brain.
Anthelmintic: Destroys or expels intestinal worms.
Antacid: Neutralizes excess stomach and intestinal acids.
Antiallergenic: Inactivates allergenic substances in the body.
Antibacterial/Antibiotic: Helps the body fight off harmful bacteria.
Antidepressant: Helps maintain emotional stability.
Anticatarrhal: Eliminates or counteracts the formation of mucus.
Anticoagulant: Thins blood and helps prevent blood clots.
Antifungal: Kills infection-causing fungi.
Anti-inflammatory: Reduces swelling of the tissues.
Anti-itch: Deadens itching sensations.
Antimicrobial: Kills a wide range of harmful bacteria, fungi, and viruses.
Antioxidant: Fights harmful oxidation.
Antipyretic/Fever Reducer: Reduces or prevents fever.
Antiseptic: External application prevents bacterial growth on skin.
Antispasmodic: Prevents or relaxes muscle tension.
Antiviral: Helps the body fight invading viruses.
Astringent: Has a constricting or binding effect. Commonly used to treat hemorrhages, secretions and diarrhea.
Blood Coagulant: Thickens blood and aids in clotting.

Carminative: Relieves gas.

Cholagogue: Encourages the flow of bile into the small intestine.

Circulatory Stimulant: Promotes even and efficient blood circulation.

Demulcent: Soothing substance, usually mucilage, taken internally to protect injured or inflamed tissues.

Diaphoretic: Induces sweating.

Diuretic: Increases urine flow.

Emetic: Induces vomiting.

Emmenagogue: Promotes menstruation.

Emollient: Softens, soothes and protects skin.

Expectorant: Assists in expelling mucus from the lungs and throat.

Galactogogue: Increases the secretion of breast milk.

Hemostatic: Stops hemorrhaging and encourages blood coagulation.

Hepatic: Tones and strengthens the liver.

Hypotensive: Lowers abnormally elevated blood pressure.

Immune-System Stimulant: Strengthens immune system so the body can fight off invading organisms.

Laxative: Promotes bowel movements.

Lithotriptic: Helps dissolve urinary and biliary stones.

Muscle Relaxant: Loosens tight muscles and reduces muscle cramping.

Nervine: Calms tension.

Oxytocic: Stimulates uterine contractions.

Rubefacient: Increases blood flow at the surface of the skin.

Sedative: Quiets the nervous system.

Sialagogue/Digestive Aid: Promotes the flow of saliva.

Stimulant: Increases the body's energy.

Tonic: Promotes the functions of body systems.

Vasoconstrictor: Constricts blood vessels, limiting the amount of blood flowing to a particular area.

Vasodilator: Dilates blood vessels, helping to promote blood flow.

Vulnerary: Encourages wound healing by promoting cell growth and repair.

HERBAL ORGANIZATIONS

Where to go for more information:

American Botanical Council
P.O. Box 201660
Austin, TX 78720
512-331-8868
www.herbalgram.org

The American Herbalist Guild
P.O. Box 746555
Arvada, CO 80006
303-423-8800

American Herbalists Guild
Box 1683
Soquel, CA 95073
408-464-2441

Herb Research Foundation
1007 Pearl Street, Suite 200
Boulder, CO 80302
303-449-2265
www.herbs.org

**National Accupuncture and
Oriental Medicine Alliance**
14637 Starr Road SE
Olalla, WA 98359
206-851-6896

**National Institutes of Health
Office of Alternative Medicine**
9000 Rockville Pike
Building 31, Room 5B-37
Mailstop 2182
Bethesda, MD 20892
301-402-2466

The Herb Society of America
9019 Kirtland-Chardon Road
Kirtland, OH 44094
216-256-0514

American College of Sports Medicine
P.O. Box 1440
Indianapolis, IN 46206
317-637-9200

American Heart Association
7272 Greenville Avenue
Dallas, TX 75231
214-373-6300

National Health Information Center
P.O. Box 1133
Washington, DC 20013
800-336-4797

GROWING HERBS

Interested in cultivating herbs yourself?
These sources can supply roots, plants and/or seeds.

Catoctin Mountain Botanicals
P.O. Box 454
Jefferson, MD 21755
301-473-4351

Companion Plants
7247 N. Coolville Ridge Rd.
Athens, OH 45701
614-593-3092
E-mail: complants@frognet.net

Dry Fork Herb Gardens
R.R.#1 Box 21
Rockport, IL
217-437-5281

Ecofriendly Farms
15488 Barn Rock Rd.
Mendota, VA 24270
540-466-8689

Goodwin Creek Gardens
P.O. Box 83
Williams, OR 97544
541-846-7357

Herbal Exchange
P.O. Box 429
9160 Lentz Rd.
Frazeysburg, OH 43822
614-828-9968

Horizon Herbs
P.O. Box 69
Williams, OR 97544
541-846-6233
www.chatlink.com/~herbseed
E-mail: herbseed@chatlink.com

Johnny's Seeds
Rt. 1 Box 2580
Foss Hill Rd.
Albion, ME 04910
207-437-9294
www.johnnyseeds.com

Mountain Traditions
H.C. 68, Box 193
Big Creek, KY 40914
606-598-6904

Nature's Cathedral
Rt. 1 Box 120
Blairstown, IA 52209
319-454-6959

Prairie Moon Nursery
Rt. 3, Box 163
Winona, MN 55987
507-452-1362

Wilcox Natural Products
P.O. Box 391
755 George Wilson Rd.
Boone, NC 28607
828-264-3615
www.goldenseal.com

Wild Wonderful Farm, Inc.
P.O. Box 256
Franklin, WV 26268
212-736-1467

INDEX

ABOUT THE AUTHOR

Stephanie Pedersen is a writer and editor who specializes in the area of health. Her articles have appeared in numerous publications, including *American Woman, Sassy, Teen, Weight Watchers* and *Woman's World*. She has also co-written *What Your Cat is Trying to Tell You: A Head-to-Tail Guide to Your Cat's Symptoms and Their Solutions* and *What Your Dog is Trying to Tell You: A Head-to-Tail Guide to Your Dog's Symptoms and Their Solutions,* both published by St. Martin's Press. She currently resides in New York City.

Picture Credits: Steve Gorton, David Murray, Dave King, Martin Norris, Philip Gatward, Andy Crawford, Philip Dowell, Clive Streeter, Peter Chadwick, Tim Ridley, Andrew Whittack, Martin Cameron

DORLING KINDERSLEY PUBLISHING, INC.
www.dk.com

Published in the United States by
Dorling Kindersley Publishing, Inc.
95 Madison Avenue • New York, New York 10016

Copyright © 2000 by Dorling Kindersley Publishing, Inc.

Editorial Director: LaVonne Carlson
Editors: Nancy Burke, Barbara Minton, Connie Robinson
Designer: Carol Wells
Cover Designer: Gus Yoo

Pedersen, Stephanie.
    Echinacea : amazing immunity / by Stephanie Pedersen.
        p.cm. -- (Natural care library)
        ISBN 0-7894-5199-9 (pb. : alk. paper)
        1.Echinacea (Plants)--Therapeutic use. I. Title. II. Series.
RS165.E4 P43 2000
615'. 32399 21--dc21
99-040021

First American Edition 1999   2 4 6 8 10 9 7 5 3